The Family Medical History Journal

I0096500

A Step-By-Step Guide to Documenting Your Family's Health History

The Family Medical History Journal

Linda Cheryl Conley McCray

Primix Publishing
11620 Wilshire Blvd
Suite 900, West Wilshire Center, Los Angeles, CA, 90025
www.primixpublishing.com
Phone: 1-800-538-5788

© 2022 Linda Cheryl Conley McCray. All rights reserved.

No part of this book may be reproduced, stored in a retrieval system, or transmitted by any means without the written permission of the author.

Published by Primix Publishing   05/11/2022

ISBN: 978-1-955944-60-1(sc)
ISBN: 978-1-955944-61-8(e)

Any people depicted in stock imagery provided by iStock are models, and such images are being used for illustrative purposes only.

Certain stock imagery © iStock.

Because of the dynamic nature of the Internet, any web addresses or links contained in this book may have changed since publication and may no longer be valid. The views expressed in this work are solely those of the author and do not necessarily reflect the views of the publisher, and the publisher hereby disclaims any responsibility for them.

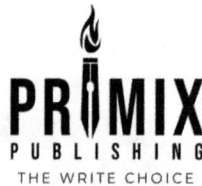

PRIMIX
PUBLISHING
THE WRITE CHOICE

This book is Recorded By

Name: _____

Date: _____

Foreword

The Family Medical Journal was created to assist families in documenting the much-needed medical histories of relatives, both living and deceased. It is imperative that family members recognize the various health problems that may exist and be problematic for future generations.

This book will serve as a great resource for documenting family medical history. There is nothing worse than being diagnosed with an ailment without knowing who else within the family may have experienced it. If a process can be implemented, allowing each person to document their medical conditions and establish a valued history, perhaps it will give future generations the knowledge they need. Our children and grandchildren will have the necessary information to assist their overall well-being.

Dedication

To my Lord and Savior, Jesus Christ, all glory, honor, and praises unto you. Thank you for allowing me another chance with this missed opportunity.

To my husband, William McCray, II, who gave me space and time to complete my thought processes in developing this book and loved me even more.

To my children, Robbie, Robert, Ty'Leece, and William III, who had medical questions, many of which I could not answer. I hope that I will be able to supply more on our health history now that I have been given better information.

To my grandchildren, Tonni, Troy, Breonna, and Ty'La, who I want to be knowledgeable about our family's health history. Please continue to document all health issues. I pray the information I have supplied regarding the four generations of our family will assist you in fighting illnesses and diseases before they become detrimental to

your health. I want you to be armed with knowledge about your family and any illnesses that may be hereditary.

To my son-in-law, Antonio Davis. I pray that you will be able to provide invaluable information for the benefit of your daughters.

To my siblings, Willie Conley, Jr., Ronald Conley, Sr., Raymond Conley, Sr., Constance Conley-Boyd, Bernard Conley, Sr., Kenneth Conley, Sr., Gary Conley, Sr., Rona Conley-Brown, and Renee Conley-Craigmiles. Thank you for all of your assistance in researching the Conley-Hawkins Family health history.

To my loving parents, Willie and Thelma Conley, who both have gone to glory. Thank you, Mom and Dad, for the wonderful ideas and views you instilled in me. Your confidence and love allowed me to know that I could accomplish anything I set my mind to.

To Betty Hawkins-Anthony and Charles Hawkins, my maternal aunt, and uncle. Thank you so much for your memories of illnesses of relatives who have passed. This knowledge has been informative.

To my first cousin, Janice Terry-Friday, I would like to thank you for your memories of family illnesses and the history of strokes in the White family health history.

To my best friend, Rainelle Edwards, who has always had an ear to hear and a shoulder to cry on.

To my wonderful and loving Pastor, Eric Mitchell, and First Lady Sheryl Mitchell, of the Greater Emmanuel Temple of Deliverance in Detroit, Michigan. Pastor, thank you for encouraging your members to utilize and develop their ideas and step out in faith to pursue their dreams. Your words of encouragement and the knowledge that you both love and support me in all of my endeavors help me feel safe.

I thank you all for your contributions to the success of this book.

Linda Cheryl Conley-McCray

January 10, 2005

Why I Wrote This Book

For over fifteen years, I worked as a Public Safety Officer for a large urban school system. My duties in this occupation included searching over 1,500 students daily, including book bags, luggage, and identification cards, ensuring the student belonged in that particular school. Of course, two or three other officers assisted me. We also had the task of stopping physical and verbal altercations, be it male or female, with one or several students, and escorting students from classes when they were disruptive.

After performing this occupation for many years, I began to notice swelling in my hands and swelling and tenderness in my shoulders. At first, the pain and swelling were random. However, the pain and swelling became more frequent as the years went by. I began experiencing painful flares to my hands. At times, one hand would be affected, and at other times, both hands would have pain. There would be tingling, numbness and burning when these incidents occurred. I could not pick up items, turn knobs, zip up, button, open jars, write, or hold a phone. I could not do everything we do with our hands that we take for granted. I could not do, even with great effort.

At times, I would fall asleep without any problems, only to awaken to sharp pain, burning, and tingling in my fingertips. The pain and ache felt as if they had their own pulse. My hands were swollen like balloons but felt heavy and cold. I could not sleep enduring that type of pain, so I would sit up, rock, and cry, unable to deal with this excruciating pain. No matter what I took, medication seemed to have no effect.

The rheumatologist I saw ran tests and placed me on medication containing cortisone (Z-Pak). My general practitioner sent me to a neurologist to find out exactly what was occurring. She did not want to give me a diagnosis until she was sure of what was wrong.

While waiting on an appointment to see the neurologist, I began experiencing difficulty lifting my arms. At first, my left shoulder would not move. A few days later, my right shoulder started to have problems. At times, the pains in my shoulders were simultaneous. The rheumatologist diagnosed tendonitis. My general practitioner gave cortisone injections in my shoulder to ease the discomfort. After so many episodes with my health, I decided it was time to return to school and pursue my master's degree. Over the next year, there were times when I would not have any problems. Then, I would have back-to-back episodes of pain. Sometimes, the pain would last for a few days. Other times, it could last five to seven days.

The visit to the neurologist's office was not anything I would wish on my worst enemy. The tests were grueling. The doctor would stick needles into my hands, wrists, forearms, shoulders, and neck. The test was administered without any medication to deaden the pain from the pins sticking into you. I was diagnosed with carpal tunnel syndrome, sent to physical therapy, and given a splint to wear. The flares of pain would continue, but not as often. As I made plans to complete my degree, which was swiftly approaching, it was a matter of time before I would be seeking a new career.

I walked across the stage at Spring Arbor University with a Master's Degree in Organizational Management on February 3, 2003. Thenext week, I went to work. My partner was absent, so a substitute was sent for the day. He was a new graduate from the police academy and had never worked in the school system. The school was fine until dismissal. Then, we had to go outside to ensure the students would clear the campus without incident.

It was cold and snowy, and the ground was covered with patches of ice. Perhaps twelve years of age, a female student stood 12 feet behind me crying. Next to her, a male student stood loudly, cursing. I responded to the female student, trying to find out what had occurred. Before I could speak to the young man, my partner for the day started wrestling with him. They both ended up on the ground. My partner was trying to put handcuffs on the young man, and a large crowd of males began to surround them. With the two of them on the ground, I knew I had to get this crowd away from them. I started to pull students away from my partner and the young man, dispersing the crowd. As I escorted the female student into the building to obtain her statement, I looked at my hands. I noticed my hands were swollen, looking like two giant balloons. They ached and were sore to the touch.

I could barely write my report, gripping the ink pen like a foreign object. My handwriting seemed messy and almost illegible, unlike my normal reports. My reports were usually neat, tidy, and precise because details were important when dealing with any in-school incident. The next day, I went to the doctor because my hands were completely swollen.

My rheumatologist took me off work, ran tests, and gave me cortisone injections in both wrists. Then he referred me to an orthopedic surgeon. The orthopedic specialist ran tests and administered another cortisone injection. We then discussed arrangements regarding the date of surgery on my wrist. I decided to put surgery off because I had already been off work for three months. I returned to work in May 2003.

On September 18, 2003, my right hand and arm swelled so largely that they looked like someone had blown them up. They were puffy and looked as if they were going to burst. Honestly, my arm looked like the Incredible Hulk's arm would have looked during transformation. When I went to the doctor, he informed me I could no longer avoid it; it was time for surgery. Prior to my carpal tunnel surgery, I began experiencing problems with my shoulders. I received cortisone injections, and the rheumatologist again referred me to the orthopedic specialist. He sent me for an MRI of my right shoulder. It was found that I had torn my rotator cuff. Two weeks later, I began experiencing the same problems with my left shoulder and was sent for an MRI of that shoulder. I had also torn my left rotator cuff.

LINDA CHERYL CONLEY MCCRAY

My Consultation With the Surgeon

The right shoulder was torn 2 ½ diameters, and after looking over the reports on both, the doctor found it the worst of the two. The orthopedic specialist decided it should be corrected first. Surgery was performed in December 2004. A pin was put into the shoulder because of the tear. I was informed that it would take approximately eight months for recovery.

In July 2005, I had surgery on my left shoulder. The procedure went well, and I was recovering. However, the second week after the surgery, I found a large knot under my left arm. It was still extremely difficult to lift this arm. My underarm felt like it was on fire. The knot under my arm was the size of a small tangerine. While I was visiting my daughter in a neighboring city, she saw the size of the knot. She immediately took me to the emergency room.

Once I arrived at the emergency room, my temperature was taken, and I was escorted to a room. When the doctor arrived, he informed me I would be staying, and a room was being prepared for me. I told the doctor I could not stay because I had a court date the following morning. I was finally going to court for my worker's compensation case, and I would not be there, according to my physician. The doctor informed me that he could not let me out of the hospital; my temperature was 105 degrees. Of course, many tests were run to find out how this situation came about, and I was placed in a private room.

The next day, a doctor that specialized in communicable diseases visited me. He informed me I was not contagious, but a surgeon would be visiting me soon to discuss how the large knot under my left arm would be handled. Later that evening, the surgeon did visit. He informed me that my white blood count was off the charts and surgery would be performed the next morning. After the surgery, I was informed that I had a bacterial infection, and it had moved in. The surgeon had to cut two plugs out of my underarm area, the size of my eyes.

It took me about 8-10 months to recover from back-to-back surgery in the same area. With more and more health issues, I grew depressed. In addition to the health problems, having no income certainly did not help the situation. I was so stressed out and unable to pay my bills I was eventually taken to the emergency room because of pain in my left side. I thought I had a heart attack. After various tests, I was released from the hospital three days later.

My rheumatoid arthritis caused me to be despondent. I was depressed because I could not complete tasks I knew I should have been able to complete. I had no initiative, nor did I have the perseverance to complete anything. The pain I was enduring did not allow me to do anything but have a pity party. I began to get back into my Bible, and I went to Bible Study. I began to have a spiritual relationship with my God. My pastor and first lady prayed for me, and I prayed for myself.

For a time, my husband had been unable to find a way to help me out of my depression. He stayed busy working regular school and night school as a teacher. He could not believe the pain I was in. However, he did have a problem with the weight I gained and told me about it. He figured that I was just having a pity party when I could not get out of bed. I was in excruciating pain, and once I took my pain medication, all I wanted to do was sleep.

When I began to feel better, I would go down to our in-home gym and work out. I did not have many of those days because the pain ruled me. All I wanted to do was eat and sleep between the Prednisone, Remicade, Methotrexate, Synthroid, Adalat, Mobic, and Premarin. I realized that I could only get through this situation one way: prayer.

I found that prayer truly changes things. I was so glad I was able to overcome my health problems. When things started looking black, I had to give the situation to God to know there was another side of through. Once I got through with all of my issues, I was able to see a light that replaced the entire three years of darkness.

The school system fired me after my three-year battle with them for worker's compensation. However, they had to pay me for everything I went through. Two weeks after receiving my check, a large firm hired me. Now, I talk on the phone instead of physically stopping fights. I am still on a lot of medication, but my stress level has eased. I do not have much money, but I can pay my bills. Thank you, God, for rescuing me.

I had so many health problems that I wanted to be assured my children and grandchildren were aware of all the issues related to me. I want them to document every health concern that may relate to them and their children. By establishing this information, my family can protect present and future generations by making them aware of any health troubles that affected us.

LINDA CHERYL CONLEY MCCRAY

ASK QUESTIONS

If you were wise enough to purchase this book, remember to ask questions. Ask questions of your grandparents, parents, aunts, uncles, cousins, and anyone else you can think of in your family tree regarding your family medical history. Write down what you can, then compile the information so that your family may be able to use it. The information found could save the lives of family members in the present and the future.

ASK

ASK

ASK

I was talking with a coworker recently. She began to tell me about her recent visit to the doctor. The doctor began by asking her questions regarding her complaints. As she described her inability to focus and make decisions, the doctor informed her she needed to look into her family history. Her physician advised her, based on everything she had told him, depression runs in her family. The doctor prescribed an anti-depressant for her. When she got home, she phoned one of her brothers, since both of her parents were deceased. She told him of her symptoms and the medication the doctor placed her on for depression. He informed her that he was placed on an anti-depressant several years ago. When she inquired why he had not mentioned it before, he stated that he did not think anything about, since he was only on the medication for a few months.

I bring up this point because, as a people, there is a tendency to be secretive about ailments.

We could question family members who should be aware of any medical problems. It is like pulling teeth to get them to disclose necessary information that could be essential to other family members.

Another Scenario

A close friend of my husband and I had to have a biopsy of her breasts. After the surgery, while talking with a female relative, she was informed, "breast cancer runs in our family." She was appalled by this news. She had asked various family members if cancer was an issue their family shared. No one was able to tell her anything. After this excruciating surgery, she was told that breast cancer runs within her family. Before the surgery, she had informed her physician that there was no cancer within her family. Therefore, biopsy surgery was necessary to detect if breast cancer was present.

Two days after having a biopsy done, she found out that several relatives on her father's side of the family had mastectomies. This lack of information is another reason for us, as a people, to begin to question elderly family members to find out as much as possible about every medical issue that may plague our families. Because of a lack of knowledge, this woman underwent a painful procedure that may not have been necessary if she had known of her family medical history.

My husband revealed that his friend had sleep apnea a few days ago. Once my husband heard this, he told his friend that he had sleep apnea as well. His friend asked my husband why he had never shared this with him previously. My husband's response: "I didn't think about it." That statement is just how we, as a people, tend to keep ailments and illnesses under wraps, like they should be secret.

Health issues should not be taboo, especially between family and friends. So, speak of these issues not for sympathy or empathy but because the information disclosed may save lives. Take the test, ask questions and be ready to record vital medical problems within the family. This activity may prove to be an education you never thought to receive. Once you get started, you may find so many symptoms, ailments, illnesses, and surgeries that you never knew about and may have occurred right under your nose. By comparing notes with other family members, you may learn someone you love is enduring some of the same symptoms that have just been documented. I cannot say this enough: ask, ask, ask, and record, record, record. Doing so may save your life or the life of someone you love.

LINDA CHERYL CONLEY MCCRAY

Reflections

In February 2003, I was injured while assisting my partner, who was trying to handcuff a student. They were both on the ground, wrestling on the ice, while 20 or more male students surrounded them. This was a dangerous situation in the making, so I began to pull one male student at a time away from this circle. After completing this task, I found both of my hands swollen.

I visited my doctor the next day, and after several months of tests and injections, I was diagnosed with carpal tunnel syndrome. I began having periods where my hands would swell, so they began to look like balloons. At that point, my rheumatologist informed me I had rheumatoid arthritis in both of my hands. The x-rays revealed nodules on the bones, and I began receiving steroid injections. The doctor prescribed a regimen of medication, including Methotrexate, Prednisone, and Plaquenil.

After I began receiving medical treatment for my rheumatoid arthritis, my physician suggested I see an ophthalmologist. One of the medications prescribed for me, although effective for arthritis treatment, could cause a problem with my eyes. Once the ophthalmologist looked over my medications, I was removed off Plaquenil. I was informed that Plaquenil attacks the macular, which is responsible for focusing the central vision in the eye. The macular also controls the ability to read, drive a car, recognize faces and colors, and see objects in fine detail. At this time, I was informed that I had macular degeneration. This caused me to reflect back 30 years ago.

I woke up one morning and could not see. I was literally blind. I had not done anything different the previous evening getting ready for bed. I had not hurt my eyes and had no other problems before this incident, which would cause me to lose my vision. Yet, I lost my sight. My husband tried to comfort me, but there was little he could do to alleviate my pain and confusion. With my eyes closed, I could feel pain and a burning sensation. My husband took me to an ophthalmologist.

I was in so much pain the doctor could hardly even examine me. The light shining in my eyes caused such unbearable pain that all I could do was scream. The doctor could not tell me what had happened to my eyes or why I could not see. He did not prescribe any medications, run any tests, or, more importantly, answer why this had happened to me. I went home, got down on my hands and knees, and prayed that God would restore my sight. Three weeks later, just as quickly as I lost my sight, I got it back.

I talked with my two daughters about their experience when I lost my sight. My eldest daughter remembered it vividly because she had an angora sweater on the washer for me to wash. Her father, being helpful, washed it because I could not perform the duties I would have normally handled. She brought the sweater upstairs when she found it was large enough to fit her Barbie. My baby girl's memory was I could not comb her hair the way she was accustomed. She did not look like the princess I always made her look like when I did her hair. I did not suffer alone when I lost my sight. Whether their memories were vain or not they also suffered when I could not see in their minds.

A few months before my mother made her transition, she began experiencing problems with her eyesight. One evening, we were visiting another church. My mother and brother were sitting in the middle aisle while I sat maybe three feet away to their right. I went over to speak to them, and my mother could not even see me. I asked her if she saw me waving at her from the other side of the church. She acknowledged she saw someone waving but was not aware it was I. I wonder if my mother was experiencing macular degeneration.

As I look back over my life and family history, I remember my dad could not sleep in the bed. If he lay in the bed, he would wake up coughing and choking. Therefore, he would fall asleep at the dining room table. While sitting there, he would snore loudly, cough, and would stop breathing. Suddenly, he would awaken and begin all over again. Based on all of the information I have gathered, what I just described could only be attributed to sleep apnea.

I was a new grandmother and responsible for picking up my new grandbaby from the east side of Detroit. I did not remember until I had gotten off of work and had to take East 8 Mile Road to my niece's home. This was a different route than I usually take, so I hit traffic. I preceded towards the railroad tracks, and as luck would have it, a train was holding up traffic. While waiting for the train to cross, which seemed to take forever, I unknowingly fell asleep. There were no cars on the east side of 8 Mile Road when I awoke. I am not even sure how long I have been sleeping. The entire situation frightened me, so I immediately called for an appointment with my general practitioner.

Once I got to my physician's office, I described what had occurred, and how tired I was after eight hours of sleep. I also informed him of my husband's description of my loud snoring and how I would stop breathing several times during the night. My general practitioner sent me to a board certified physician who specialized in sleep/pulmonary medicine. A sleep study was conducted and concluded that I stopped breathing over seventy times throughout the night. The doctor prescribed a C-PAP machine. I began sleeping with a mask that pumped the air as I slept. Now, I feel rested instead of tired after a night's sleep. As I reflect, I see all of the ailments I have been diagnosed with, many I had no idea fit into my family health history.

The ailments I believed I would be susceptible to are diabetes, hypertension and gallbladder problems since both of my parents had to have gallbladder surgery in their 50s and 60s. My sister, Connie, had gallbladder surgery at the age of 23. My brother, Kenny, had gallbladder surgery at the age of 22. Both went through surgery without any incidents. I had gallbladder surgery at the age of 26. I was admitted into the hospital on October 1, 1979. I was admitted early for tests to be run. On October 7, 1979, my surgery was performed. The day after surgery, the nursing staff got me up to walk around. I had two holes in my stomach. One was described as the drainage hole, and the other was a large scar about seven inches above the drainage hole. I was able to walk for two days straight, but I just could not get out of bed on the third day.

The surgeon who performed the procedure came to see me and, after checking me over, told me I looked swollen. He asked me at the time if I was pregnant. I could not believe he would ask me that, considering the reason I checked into the hospital a week early was so that blood and urine tests could be conducted. My birth control pills were on the nightstand. I told him that I had not missed taking any pills. He sent the lab tech for blood to be taken. The result: I was pregnant.

Immediately after my pregnancy was confirmed, I became deathly ill. My white blood cells became elevated, my temperature rose, and I could not get out of bed. I called for a nurse, but no one came to see about me. An elderly patient I had begun to visit on my daily walk noticed my light on. He also noticed I could not get out of bed. He went straight to the nurses' station to tell them to check on me. The nurses still did not come. However, my eldest brother came to visit me about ten minutes later. He saw my light was on and observed that I looked green in color. My brother asked me how long my light had been on. I was not able to tell him, only give him an estimation. The elderly patient across the hall told him. He went up to the nurses' station. I am unsure what my brother said to the nurses, but they beat him back to my room.

The nurses checked me out and found my temperature was 104 degrees. They called a code blue, and people in white surrounded my bed. They began to pack me in ice to bring down my body temperature. I was completely unaware of what was going on for the next day. I was not released from the hospital until October 30, 1979. Even though I was pregnant, based on the trauma my body had gone through, my gynecologist performed a therapeutic abortion.

While researching our family medical history, among my siblings alone, I have found that out of 10 children, two have diabetes, six have hypertension, seven wear glasses due to astigmatism, two have hypothyroidism, and two have gout. I am the only one who has been diagnosed with rheumatoid arthritis. In the last two years, I have been prescribed Remicade, a medication that has to be infused into my bloodstream every eight weeks. As ironic as it may be, I believed I only had to be concerned with hereditary illnesses. Never in my wildest dreams did I think of being diagnosed with an ailment I had not even heard of.

My mother died at the young age of 63 of uterine cancer. Although the surgery was performed to remove the cancer, it had metastasized and spread throughout her body. In a matter of weeks, my mother was gone. Eight years later, my father died at the age of 76. He had one stroke, and then another followed the first. He developed dementia, and a few months later, Daddy was gone.

In my research of the White family medical history, I found that my paternal grandmother, Lubertha White-Conley, and my father's only sibling, Jessie Terry, also died from strokes. This is important information, helping my family explore and understand what may contribute to stroke.

My maternal grandmother, Ruby Labelle Bayman-Hawkins, died from a brain aneurysm. One of my maternal first cousins had a brain aneurysm. She was fortunate enough to have two successful surgeries. My maternal grandfather died from diabetes at the age of 41. Are strokes and aneurysms hereditary in my family? Certainly, these questions need to be further explored to gather a complete family medical history that will benefit future generations.

Ailments I Have Been Diagnosed With

Hypertension	Both
Hypothyroidism (Underactive thyroid)	Mother
Astigmatism -	Mother
Sleep apnea -	Father
Macular degeneration -	Unknown
Rheumatoid arthritis -	Unknown

Hypertension is more commonly known as high blood pressure. The cause of hypertension remains unclear, but various conditions such as lack of exercise, poor diet, obesity, genetics, etc., can lead to hypertension. The blood pressure reading is measured in millimeters of mercury. It is written as systolic pressure (the force of the blood against the artery walls as your heart beats) over diastolic pressure (the blood pressure between heartbeats).

Reading blood pressure is the same but may vary according to that person's reading. Normal blood pressure is systolic pressure less than 120 and diastolic pressure less than 80. Prehypertension is a systolic pressure of 120-139 or a diastolic pressure of 80-89. Stage 1 Hypertension is blood pressure greater than systolic pressure of 140-159 or a diastolic pressure of 90-99 or greater. Stage 2 Hypertension is a systolic pressure of 160 or greater or diastolic pressure of 100 or greater.

Hypertension does not usually have any symptoms, so one does not feel it. A healthcare professional can diagnose it during an office visit. It is crucial to be checked, especially if a close relative has hypertension or has the risk factors associated with the disease. If blood pressure is extremely high, one may have intense headaches, chest pain, and heart failure. Secondary hypertension is less common, resulting from another condition or disorder, such as kidney disease or sleep apnea. If left untreated, hypertension can be deadly. It is imperative to discover if one has hypertension to live. It can affect one's vision, heart, and kidneys and cause eye disease. Hypertension is often called a silent killer.

Treating hypertension usually involves lifestyle modifications and possibly, drug treatment. One can start exercising, losing weight, eating healthy, reducing salt intake, and limiting alcohol to assist in treatment. Hypertension medications include ACE (angiotensin-converting enzyme) inhibitors, angiotensin receptor blockers, beta-blockers, and calcium channel blockers. Some medicines being taken for another condition may cause high blood pressure. These medications include amphetamines, Ritalin, corticosteroids, hormones (including birth control pills), migraine medications, cyclosporine, and erythropoietin. One must also be careful of OTC (over-the-counter) medications, such as allergy and cold medications and appetite suppressants.

The thyroid is a butterfly shaped organ located in front of the neck, just over the windpipe. It produces hormones containing iodine, which regulate how body cells use energy and produce heat. There are two different diseases involving the thyroid. Hyperthyroidism may cause an increase in body metabolism, resulting in weight loss, regardless of appetite, excessive warmth, and sweating. The thyroid gland may also swell, causing a goiter.

The condition I have been diagnosed with is the opposite of the above. Hypothyroidism is a condition where too little hormone is secreted. Consequently, the body slows down, with symptoms including coldness, sluggishness, dry skin, and scanty hair growth. Recognizing and treating deficient production of thyroid hormone can be treated by replacing the normal amount of the chemical the body requires.

Astigmatism is an optical defect whereby vision is blurred due to an irregular curvature of the cornea. The cornea is like an egg in corneal astigmatism rather than spherical. This reduces the cornea's ability to focus light. In lenticular astigmatism, the curvature of the lens is not even, resulting in scattering rather than focusing light on the retina. When light strikes the retina at multiple points, the result is blurred vision. Astigmatism causes difficulties in seeing fine detail, and in some cases, vertical lines may appear to be leaning over. The effects of astigmatism of the eye can often be corrected with prosthetic lenses, contact lenses, or refractive surgery.

The word apnea, translated from Greek, literally means "without breath." There are three types of apnea: obstructive, central, and mixed. The most common is obstructive apnea. In all types of untreated apnea, people stop breathing repeatedly during sleep. A blockage of the airway causes obstructive apnea, usually when the soft tissue in the rear of the throat closes during sleep. The airway is not blocked in central apnea, but the brain fails to signal the muscles to breathe. Mixed apnea is a combination of the two. With each apnea event, the brain arouses people with sleep apnea to resume breathing, but sleep is fragmented and of poor quality.

According to the National Institute of Health, sleep apnea affects more than twelve million Americans and is very common. Risk factors include being male, overweight, and over forty. However, sleep apnea can strike anyone, at any age, even children. Yet because of a lack of awareness, many people remain undiagnosed and untreated.

Untreated sleep apnea can cause high blood pressure, memory problems, weight gain, impotence, and headaches. It may also be responsible for job impairment and motor vehicle accidents. Fortunately, sleep apnea can be diagnosed and treated with several treatment options available.

Macular degeneration is an incurable eye disease and the leading cause of blindness for those 55 and older in the United States. This disease affects more than 10 million Americans. Macular degeneration is caused by the deterioration of the retina's central portion, the inside back layer of the eye that records the images we see and sends them to the brain. The retina's central portion, known as the macula, is responsible for focusing central vision in the eye. It also controls our ability to read, drive a car, recognize faces or colors, and see objects in fine detail. As people age, their chances of developing eye diseases increase. Unfortunately, the causes of macular degeneration are not conclusively known. Research into this disease is limited by insufficient funding.

The cause of rheumatoid arthritis (also known as R A) is unknown and studied throughout the scientific arena. It is believed by some scientists that R A is genetically inherited. R A may also trigger the immune system to attack the body's own tissues, which results in inflammation throughout various areas of the body, including the lungs and eyes.

Symptoms of rheumatoid arthritis may come and go. When there is inflammation in the body, the disease is active. Remission occurs when inflammation subsides and can last for weeks, months, or years. Symptoms can include fatigue, lack of appetite, low-grade fever, stiffness, and muscle and joint aches when the disease is active. The stiffness is typically most notable in the morning or after long periods of inactivity. Arthritis is common at this time, along with swollen, tender, painful joints.

R A is a systemic disease, meaning the inflammation can affect organs, and the joints. Chronic inflammation can cause damage to body tissues, cartilage, and bone. This leads to loss of cartilage, erosion, and weakness of the bones and muscles, which may lead to a loss of function.

R A can even affect the joint responsible for tightening vocal cords in rare instances. This may change the tone of the voice, causing hoarseness.

Medications I Take

Premarin for Hormone Replacement

Adalat for Hypertension

Methotrexate for Rheumatoid Arthritis (R A)

Mobic for Rheumatoid Arthritis (R A)

Predisone for Rheumatoid Arthritis (R A)

Remicade forRheumatoid Arthritis (R A)

Synthroid for Under active thyroid

Premarin is a mixture of estrogen hormones used to treat symptoms of menopause, such as hot flashes, vaginal burning, drying, and irritation. The medication may prevent osteoporosis in women who have gone through menopause and ovarian failure in others. Premarin may also be used as part of cancer treatment in men and women. This medication is not recommended for people who have heart conditions, liver disease, or hormone-related cancers. Long-term use may increase the chance of developing breast cancer, heart attack, stroke, or endometrial hyperplasia (a condition that may lead to cancer of the uterus).

Adalat is in a class of drugs called calcium channel blockers. This drug is used to widen (relax) the blood vessels, making it easier for the heart to pump and reduce its workload. In other words, this medication is used to lower hypertension or treat angina. One should avoid drinking grapefruit juice or eating grapefruit when using this medication.

Methotrexate is one of the most effective and commonly used medicines to treat arthritis and other rheumatic conditions. It is known as a DMARD, or a disease-modifying anti-rheumatic drug because it decreases pain and swelling and reduces joint damage. This medication was previously used for psoriasis and forms of cancer. It gained approval by the FDA for rheumatic conditions in 1988. Methotrexate blocks the production of enzymes associated with folic acid, cells comprised of growing skin, blood, and the immune system.

Mobic (meloxicam) is an NSAID, a non-steroid anti-inflammatory drug. Typically, NSAIDs are used to treat pain and inflammation. Meloxicam blocks the enzymes that contribute to pain, tenderness, and swelling associated with osteoarthritis and rheumatoid arthritis.

Prednisone, a corticosteroid, is similar to hormones produced by the body's adrenal glands. This medication replaces hormones when the body does not make enough of them, promoting its healing powers. Prednisone relieves inflammation, heat, redness, and pain associated with arthritis. It may also be used for specific thyroid and intestinal disorders, allergies, and asthma. This medication is also considered an NSAID, blocking the pathways that cause swelling.

Remicade is given by IV infusion, which generally takes about two hours. A healthcare professional in a supervised environment must administer this medication. The process of receiving the medication takes three steps. First, one has to be weighed by a nurse, or nurse's aide, to calculate the dosage of Remicade to be received. A patient's blood pressure, pulse, and temperature are also taken to ensure all is normal before the process begins. IV placement is the second step, with the health professional placing the IV in the arm while the patient sits comfortably. The last step is to merely relax while the infusion takes place. The nurse or aide checks on the patient to make sure everything is going accordingly.

Allergies

Allergic reactions can be just as deadly as illnesses one may not know about. As a 16-year-old, I found out the hard way that an allergic reaction to medication could cause harm. I was sick, vomiting, and running a high fever. This went on for several days, eventually getting to where I could not even lift my head. My parents rushed me to the emergency room.

The hospital ran tests to find out what was wrong. The general practitioner called in a gynecologist. He informed my parents I was pregnant and throwing up my stomach. My white blood count was high, and I had an infection. I was given an antibiotic, penicillin. Immediately, my esophagus began to swell. If I had not already been in the hospital being watched, I would have died.

Antibiotics are medications frequently used to prevent bacterial infections, including strep throat and ear infections. Penicillin and its family of antibiotics are used every day and can be taken orally or injected. Most people can take antibiotics without any difficulty. However, for others, antibiotics are dangerous. A penicillin allergy can develop over time, triggering an allergic reaction.

Penicillin allergy is one of the most common, including rash, hives, itchy eyes, and swollen lips, tongue, or face. However, more severe reactions can occur, resulting in an anaphylactic response. This can cause airways to swell, with wheezing, lightheadedness, slurred speech, weak pulse, nausea, diarrhea, and blueness of the skin.

Allergies

Name of medication:_____

Type of allergy:_____

Signs & Symptoms:_____

_____

_____

_____

_____

_____

Treatment: _____

_____

_____

_____

_____

_____

LINDA CHERYL CONLEY MCCRAY

Illnesses to Be On the Lookout For (My Family)

Aneurysms & Strokes

An aneurysm is an enlargement of a wall of blood vessels, usually caused by hypertension and trauma, infection, or a congenital weakness in the vessel wall. Aneurysms are significant in the aorta but can also occur in the lower extremities of older people or the intracranial area. Many aneurysms are present without symptoms, only discovered by feeling or x-ray during routine exams. When symptoms occur, they could include a pulsing sensation and pain. Symptoms of an aneurysm depend on its location. For example, if the aneurysm is in the chest, there may be pain in the upper back, difficulty in swallowing, coughing, and hoarseness.

A ruptured aneurysm can produce sudden and severe pain and, depending on the location and amount of bleeding can cause shock, loss of consciousness, and death. In most cases, emergency surgery is necessary to stop the bleeding. Clots may form in the aneurysm, creating the danger of embolisms in organs.

Aneurysms can be diagnosed through angiograms, an x-ray of the arteries, veins, or heart chambers. This x-ray may be obtained by injecting dye into the bloodstream to make them more visible. In some instances, an MRI (magnetic resonance imaging) can be used to spot an aneurysm. An echocardiogram, which uses ultrasound waves to visualize the heart chambers, and an x-ray can also be used to diagnose an aneurysm.

Congenital aneurysms cannot be prevented. A healthy lifestyle can help prevent or slow down conditions that may cause aneurysms. Hypertension should be carefully controlled to avoid aneurysm formation or extension. Hypertension also plays a factor in heart attacks and stroke. With heart attack and stroke victims, every second counts. When it happens, it is a life-and-death situation. If one has any symptoms, immediately call 9-1-1.

Coronary heart disease is America's number one killer, with stroke being number three on the list and a leading cause of disability. Based on this information, it is easy to see why risk factors must be reduced. Some heart attacks are sudden, with no doubt of what's happening. Others, however, are not so evident. One may experience chest discomfort or pain in the back, neck, jaw, stomach, or one or both arms. There may be shortness of breath, nausea, and lightheadedness. It is important to learn the signs to decrease the number of people who die or become disabled from these two diseases.

Stroke warning signs include sudden numbness or weakness of the face, arm, or leg, especially on one side of the body, sudden trouble speaking andunderstanding, confusion, dizziness, and headache without cause. Remember, time is of the essence, so immediately call emergency medical service personnel if someone experiences the above symptoms. Also, check the time the symptoms initially appeared. If certain medications are given within three hours of onset, then long-term disability can be avoided for certain types of stroke.

LINDA CHERYL CONLEY MCCRAY

My List of Medications & Ailment

Medication   Ailment

DOCUMENTING YOUR FAMILY MEDICAL HISTORY

Contents

All About Me 25

    About My Children 28

    About My Siblings 40

    About My Mother 55

    About My Maternal Grandmother 56

    About My Maternal Grandfather 57

    About My Mother's Siblings 58

All About My Paternal Family 69

    About My Father 70

    About My Paternal Grandmother 71

    About My Paternal Grandfather 72

    About My Father's Siblings 73

All About My Spouse's Family 83

    All About My Spouse 85

    About His/Her Siblings 86

About My Spouse's Maternal Family 97

    About His/Her Mother 99

    About His/Her Maternal Grandmother 100

    About His/Her Maternal Grandfather 101

    About His/Her Mother's Siblings 102

About My Spouse's Paternal Family 113

    About His/Her Father 115

About His/Her Paternal Grandmother 116

About His/Her Paternal Grandfather 117

About His/Her Father's Siblings 118

Stories That Touched My Life 129

ALL ABOUT ME

All About Me

Full Name: _____

    Maiden Name: _____

Date of Birth: _____

Place of Birth: _____

Types of childhood illnesses I experienced: _____

_____

Types of adult illnesses I experienced: _____

_____

Blood Type: _____ Allergies: _____

_____

Weight: _____ Height: _____ Eyeglasses: _____

Surgeries: _____

Age When Died: _____ Date of Death: _____

Cause of Death: _____

_____

Where buried: _____

_____

Children: _____

_____

_____

About My Children

Full Name: _____

Maiden Name: _____

Date of Birth: _____

Place of Birth: _____

Types of childhood illnesses I experienced: _____

_____

Types of adult illnesses I experienced: _____

_____

Blood Type: _____ Allergies: _____

_____

Weight: _____ Height: _____ Eyeglasses: _____

Surgeries: _____

Age When Died: _____ Date of Death: _____

Cause of Death: _____

_____

Where buried: _____

_____

Children: _____

_____

_____

Full Name: _____

    Maiden Name: _____

Date of Birth: _____

Place of Birth: _____

Types of childhood illnesses I experienced: _____

_____

Types of adult illnesses I experienced: _____

_____

Blood Type: _____ Allergies: _____

_____

Weight: _____ Height: _____ Eyeglasses: _____

Surgeries: _____

Age When Died: _____ Date of Death: _____

Cause of Death: _____

_____

Where buried: _____

_____

Children: _____

_____

_____

Full Name: _____

    Maiden Name: _____

Date of Birth: _____

Place of Birth: _____

Types of childhood illnesses I experienced: _____

_____

Types of adult illnesses I experienced: _____

_____

Blood Type: _____ Allergies: _____

_____

Weight: _____ Height: _____ Eyeglasses: _____

Surgeries: _____

Age When Died: _____ Date of Death: _____

Cause of Death: _____

_____

Where buried: _____

_____

Children: _____

_____

_____

Full Name: _____

    Maiden Name: _____

Date of Birth: _____

Place of Birth: _____

Types of childhood illnesses I experienced: _____

_____

Types of adult illnesses I experienced: _____

_____

Blood Type: _____ Allergies: _____

_____

Weight: _____ Height: _____ Eyeglasses: _____

Surgeries: _____

Age When Died: _____ Date of Death: _____

Cause of Death: _____

_____

Where buried: _____

_____

Children: _____

_____

_____

Full Name: _____

Maiden Name: _____

Date of Birth: _____

Place of Birth: _____

Types of childhood illnesses I experienced: _____

_____

Types of adult illnesses I experienced: _____

_____

Blood Type: _____ Allergies: _____

_____

Weight: _____ Height: _____ Eyeglasses: _____

Surgeries: _____

Age When Died: _____ Date of Death: _____

Cause of Death: _____

_____

Where buried: _____

_____

Children:_____

_____

_____

LINDA CHERYL CONLEY MCCRAY

Full Name: _____

    Maiden Name: _____

Date of Birth: _____

Place of Birth: _____

Types of childhood illnesses I experienced: _____

_____

Types of adult illnesses I experienced: _____

_____

Blood Type: _____ Allergies: _____

_____

Weight: _____ Height: _____ Eyeglasses: _____

Surgeries: _____

Age When Died: _____ Date of Death: _____

Cause of Death: _____

_____

Where buried: _____

_____

Children: _____

_____

_____

Full Name: _____

    Maiden Name: _____

Date of Birth: _____

Place of Birth: _____

Types of childhood illnesses I experienced: _____

_____

Types of adult illnesses I experienced: _____

_____

Blood Type: _____ Allergies: _____

_____

Weight: _____ Height: _____ Eyeglasses: _____

Surgeries: _____

Age When Died: _____ Date of Death: _____

Cause of Death: _____

_____

Where buried: _____

_____

Children: _____

_____

_____

Full Name: _____

    Maiden Name: _____

Date of Birth: _____

Place of Birth: _____

Types of childhood illnesses I experienced: _____

_____

Types of adult illnesses I experienced: _____

_____

Blood Type: _____   Allergies: _____

_____

Weight: _____   Height: _____   Eyeglasses: _____

Surgeries: _____

Age When Died: _____   Date of Death: _____

Cause of Death: _____

_____

Where buried: _____

_____

Children: _____

_____

_____

Full Name: _____

    Maiden Name: _____

Date of Birth: _____

Place of Birth: _____

Types of childhood illnesses I experienced: _____

_____

Types of adult illnesses I experienced: _____

_____

Blood Type: _____ Allergies: _____

_____

Weight: _____ Height: _____ Eyeglasses: _____

Surgeries: _____

Age When Died: _____ Date of Death: _____

Cause of Death: _____

_____

Where buried: _____

_____

Children:_____

_____

_____

Full Name: _____

    Maiden Name: _____

Date of Birth: _____

Place of Birth: _____

Types of childhood illnesses I experienced: _____

_____

Types of adult illnesses I experienced: _____

_____

Blood Type: _____ Allergies: _____

_____

Weight: _____ Height: _____ Eyeglasses: _____

Surgeries: _____

Age When Died: _____ Date of Death: _____

Cause of Death: _____

_____

Where buried: _____

_____

Children:_____

_____

_____

Full Name: _____

    Maiden Name: _____

Date of Birth: _____

Place of Birth: _____

Types of childhood illnesses I experienced: _____

_____

Types of adult illnesses I experienced: _____

_____

Blood Type: _____ Allergies: _____

_____

Weight: _____ Height: _____ Eyeglasses: _____

Surgeries: _____

Age When Died: _____ Date of Death: _____

Cause of Death: _____

_____

Where buried: _____

_____

Children: _____

_____

_____

Full Name: _____

Maiden Name: _____

Date of Birth: _____

Place of Birth: _____

Types of childhood illnesses I experienced: _____

_____

Types of adult illnesses I experienced: _____

_____

Blood Type: _____   Allergies: _____

_____

Weight: _____   Height: _____   Eyeglasses: _____

Surgeries: _____

Age When Died: _____   Date of Death: _____

Cause of Death: _____

_____

Where buried: _____

_____

Children: _____

_____

_____

About My Siblings

Full Name: _____

    Maiden Name: _____

Date of Birth: _____

Place of Birth: _____

Types of childhood illnesses I experienced: _____

_____

Types of adult illnesses I experienced: _____

_____

Blood Type: _____ Allergies: _____

_____

Weight: _____ Height: _____ Eyeglasses: _____

Surgeries: _____

Age When Died: _____ Date of Death: _____

Cause of Death: _____

_____

Where buried: _____

_____

Children: _____

_____

_____

Full Name: _____

    Maiden Name: _____

Date of Birth: _____

Place of Birth: _____

Types of childhood illnesses I experienced: _____

_____

Types of adult illnesses I experienced: _____

_____

Blood Type: _____   Allergies: _____

_____

Weight: _____   Height: _____   Eyeglasses: _____

Surgeries: _____

Age When Died: _____   Date of Death: _____

Cause of Death: _____

_____

Where buried: _____

_____

Children: _____

_____

_____

Full Name: _____

    Maiden Name: _____

Date of Birth: _____

Place of Birth: _____

Types of childhood illnesses I experienced: _____

_____

Types of adult illnesses I experienced: _____

_____

Blood Type: _____   Allergies: _____

_____

Weight: _____   Height: _____   Eyeglasses: _____

Surgeries: _____

Age When Died: _____   Date of Death: _____

Cause of Death: _____

_____

Where buried: _____

_____

Children: _____

_____

_____

Full Name: _____

    Maiden Name: _____

Date of Birth: _____

Place of Birth: _____

Types of childhood illnesses I experienced: _____

_____

Types of adult illnesses I experienced: _____

_____

Blood Type: _____ Allergies: _____

_____

Weight: _____ Height: _____ Eyeglasses: _____

Surgeries: _____

Age When Died: _____ Date of Death: _____

Cause of Death: _____

_____

Where buried: _____

_____

Children: _____

_____

_____

Full Name: _____

Maiden Name: _____

Date of Birth: _____

Place of Birth: _____

Types of childhood illnesses I experienced: _____

_____

Types of adult illnesses I experienced: _____

_____

Blood Type: _____   Allergies: _____

_____

Weight: _____   Height: _____   Eyeglasses: _____

Surgeries: _____

Age When Died: _____   Date of Death: _____

Cause of Death: _____

_____

Where buried: _____

_____

Children: _____

_____

_____

Full Name: _____

    Maiden Name: _____

Date of Birth: _____

Place of Birth: _____

Types of childhood illnesses I experienced: _____
_____

Types of adult illnesses I experienced: _____
_____

Blood Type: _____   Allergies: _____
_____

Weight: _____   Height: _____   Eyeglasses: _____

Surgeries: _____

Age When Died: _____   Date of Death: _____

Cause of Death: _____
_____

Where buried: _____
_____

Children: _____
_____
_____

Full Name: _____

    Maiden Name: _____

Date of Birth: _____

Place of Birth: _____

Types of childhood illnesses I experienced: _____

_____

Types of adult illnesses I experienced: _____

_____

Blood Type: _____   Allergies: _____

_____

Weight: _____   Height: _____   Eyeglasses: _____

Surgeries: _____

Age When Died: _____   Date of Death: _____

Cause of Death: _____

_____

Where buried: _____

_____

Children: _____

_____

_____

Full Name: _____

    Maiden Name: _____

Date of Birth: _____

Place of Birth: _____

Types of childhood illnesses I experienced: _____

_____

Types of adult illnesses I experienced: _____

_____

Blood Type: _____ Allergies: _____

_____

Weight: _____ Height: _____ Eyeglasses: _____

Surgeries: _____

Age When Died: _____ Date of Death: _____

Cause of Death: _____

_____

Where buried: _____

_____

Children: _____

_____

_____

Full Name: _____

    Maiden Name: _____

Date of Birth: _____

Place of Birth: _____

Types of childhood illnesses I experienced: _____

_____

Types of adult illnesses I experienced: _____

_____

Blood Type: _____   Allergies: _____

_____

Weight: _____   Height: _____   Eyeglasses: _____

Surgeries: _____

Age When Died: _____   Date of Death: _____

Cause of Death: _____

_____

Where buried: _____

_____

Children: _____

_____

_____

LINDA CHERYL CONLEY MCCRAY

Full Name: _____

    Maiden Name: _____

Date of Birth: _____

Place of Birth: _____

Types of childhood illnesses I experienced: _____

_____

Types of adult illnesses I experienced: _____

_____

Blood Type: _____   Allergies: _____

_____

Weight: _____   Height: _____   Eyeglasses: _____

Surgeries: _____

Age When Died: _____   Date of Death: _____

Cause of Death: _____

_____

Where buried: _____

_____

Children: _____

_____

_____

Full Name: _____

    Maiden Name: _____

Date of Birth: _____

Place of Birth: _____

Types of childhood illnesses I experienced: _____

_____

Types of adult illnesses I experienced: _____

_____

Blood Type: _____ Allergies: _____

_____

Weight: _____ Height: _____ Eyeglasses: _____

Surgeries: _____

Age When Died: _____ Date of Death: _____

Cause of Death: _____

_____

Where buried: _____

_____

Children:_____

_____

_____

Full Name: _____

    Maiden Name: _____

Date of Birth: _____

Place of Birth: _____

Types of childhood illnesses I experienced: _____
_____

Types of adult illnesses I experienced: _____
_____

Blood Type: _____ Allergies: _____
_____

Weight: _____ Height: _____ Eyeglasses: _____

Surgeries: _____

Age When Died: _____ Date of Death: _____

Cause of Death: _____
_____

Where buried: _____
_____

Children: _____
_____
_____

ALL ABOUT MY MATERNAL FAMILY

About My Mother

Full Name: _____

    Maiden Name: _____

Date of Birth: _____

Place of Birth: _____

Types of childhood illnesses I experienced: _____
_____

Types of adult illnesses I experienced: _____
_____

Blood Type: _____ Allergies: _____
_____

Weight: _____ Height: _____ Eyeglasses: _____

Surgeries: _____

Age When Died: _____ Date of Death: _____

Cause of Death: _____
_____

Where buried: _____
_____

Children: _____
_____
_____

About My Maternal Grandmother

Full Name: _____

    Maiden Name: _____

Date of Birth: _____

Place of Birth: _____

Types of childhood illnesses I experienced: _____

_____

Types of adult illnesses I experienced: _____

_____

Blood Type: _____ Allergies: _____

_____

Weight: _____ Height: _____ Eyeglasses: _____

Surgeries: _____

Age When Died: _____ Date of Death: _____

Cause of Death: _____

_____

Where buried: _____

_____

Children: _____

_____

_____

About My Maternal Grandfather

Full Name: _____

    Maiden Name: _____

Date of Birth: _____

Place of Birth: _____

Types of childhood illnesses I experienced: _____

_____

Types of adult illnesses I experienced: _____

_____

Blood Type: _____ Allergies: _____

_____

Weight: _____ Height: _____ Eyeglasses: _____

Surgeries: _____

Age When Died: _____ Date of Death: _____

Cause of Death: _____

_____

Where buried: _____

_____

Children: _____

_____

_____

About My Mother's Siblings

Full Name: _____

    Maiden Name: _____

Date of Birth: _____

Place of Birth: _____

Types of childhood illnesses I experienced: _____

_____

Types of adult illnesses I experienced: _____

_____

Blood Type: _____ Allergies: _____

_____

Weight: _____ Height: _____ Eyeglasses: _____

Surgeries: _____

Age When Died: _____ Date of Death: _____

Cause of Death: _____

_____

Where buried: _____

_____

Children: _____

_____

_____

Full Name: _____

    Maiden Name: _____

Date of Birth: _____

Place of Birth: _____

Types of childhood illnesses I experienced: _____

_____

Types of adult illnesses I experienced: _____

_____

Blood Type: _____ Allergies: _____

_____

Weight: _____ Height: _____ Eyeglasses: _____

Surgeries: _____

Age When Died: _____ Date of Death: _____

Cause of Death: _____

_____

Where buried: _____

_____

Children: _____

_____

_____

Full Name: _____

    Maiden Name: _____

Date of Birth: _____

Place of Birth: _____

Types of childhood illnesses I experienced: _____

_____

Types of adult illnesses I experienced: _____

_____

Blood Type: _____ Allergies: _____

_____

Weight: _____ Height: _____ Eyeglasses: _____

Surgeries: _____

Age When Died: _____ Date of Death: _____

Cause of Death: _____

_____

Where buried: _____

_____

Children: _____

_____

_____

Full Name: _____

Maiden Name: _____

Date of Birth: _____

Place of Birth: _____

Types of childhood illnesses I experienced: _____

_____

Types of adult illnesses I experienced: _____

_____

Blood Type: _____   Allergies: _____

_____

Weight: _____   Height: _____   Eyeglasses: _____

Surgeries: _____

Age When Died: _____   Date of Death: _____

Cause of Death: _____

_____

Where buried: _____

_____

Children: _____

_____

_____

Full Name: _____

   Maiden Name: _____

Date of Birth: _____

Place of Birth: _____

Types of childhood illnesses I experienced: _____

_____

Types of adult illnesses I experienced: _____

_____

Blood Type: _____ Allergies: _____

_____

Weight: _____ Height: _____ Eyeglasses: _____

Surgeries: _____

Age When Died: _____ Date of Death: _____

Cause of Death: _____

_____

Where buried: _____

_____

Children: _____

_____

_____

Full Name: _____

    Maiden Name: _____

Date of Birth: _____

Place of Birth: _____

Types of childhood illnesses I experienced: _____

_____

Types of adult illnesses I experienced: _____

_____

Blood Type: _____ Allergies: _____

_____

Weight: _____ Height: _____ Eyeglasses: _____

Surgeries: _____

Age When Died: _____ Date of Death: _____

Cause of Death: _____

_____

Where buried: _____

_____

Children:_____

_____

_____

Full Name: _____

    Maiden Name: _____

Date of Birth: _____

Place of Birth: _____

Types of childhood illnesses I experienced: _____

_____

Types of adult illnesses I experienced: _____

_____

Blood Type: _____   Allergies: _____

_____

Weight: _____   Height: _____   Eyeglasses: _____

Surgeries: _____

Age When Died: _____   Date of Death: _____

Cause of Death: _____

_____

Where buried: _____

_____

Children: _____

_____

_____

Full Name: _____

    Maiden Name: _____

Date of Birth: _____

Place of Birth: _____

Types of childhood illnesses I experienced: _____

_____

Types of adult illnesses I experienced: _____

_____

Blood Type: _____ Allergies: _____

_____

Weight: _____ Height: _____ Eyeglasses: _____

Surgeries: _____

Age When Died: _____ Date of Death: _____

Cause of Death: _____

_____

Where buried: _____

_____

Children: _____

_____

_____

Full Name: _____

    Maiden Name: _____

Date of Birth: _____

Place of Birth: _____

Types of childhood illnesses I experienced: _____

_____

Types of adult illnesses I experienced: _____

_____

Blood Type: _____   Allergies: _____

_____

Weight: _____   Height: _____   Eyeglasses: _____

Surgeries: _____

Age When Died: _____   Date of Death: _____

Cause of Death: _____

_____

Where buried: _____

_____

Children:_____

_____

_____

Full Name: _____

    Maiden Name: _____

Date of Birth: _____

Place of Birth: _____

Types of childhood illnesses I experienced: _____

_____

Types of adult illnesses I experienced: _____

_____

Blood Type: _____ Allergies: _____

_____

Weight: _____ Height: _____ Eyeglasses: _____

Surgeries: _____

Age When Died: _____ Date of Death: _____

Cause of Death: _____

_____

Where buried: _____

_____

Children: _____

_____

_____

ALL ABOUT MY PATERNAL FAMILY

About My Father

Full Name: _____

     Maiden Name: _____

Date of Birth: _____

Place of Birth: _____

Types of childhood illnesses I experienced: _____

_____

Types of adult illnesses I experienced: _____

_____

Blood Type: _____ Allergies: _____

_____

Weight: _____ Height: _____ Eyeglasses: _____

Surgeries: _____

Age When Died: _____ Date of Death: _____

Cause of Death: _____

_____

Where buried: _____

_____

Children: _____

_____

_____

About My Paternal Grandmother

Full Name: _____

    Maiden Name: _____

Date of Birth: _____

Place of Birth: _____

Types of childhood illnesses I experienced: _____

_____

Types of adult illnesses I experienced: _____

_____

Blood Type: _____ Allergies: _____

_____

Weight: _____ Height: _____ Eyeglasses: _____

Surgeries: _____

Age When Died: _____ Date of Death: _____

Cause of Death: _____

_____

Where buried: _____

_____

Children: _____

_____

_____

About My Paternal Grandfather

Full Name: _____

    Maiden Name: _____

Date of Birth: _____

Place of Birth: _____

Types of childhood illnesses I experienced: _____

_____

Types of adult illnesses I experienced: _____

_____

Blood Type: _____ Allergies: _____

_____

Weight: _____ Height: _____ Eyeglasses: _____

Surgeries: _____

Age When Died: _____ Date of Death: _____

Cause of Death: _____

_____

Where buried: _____

_____

Children: _____

_____

_____

About My Father's Siblings

Full Name: _____

    Maiden Name: _____

Date of Birth: _____

Place of Birth: _____

Types of childhood illnesses I experienced: _____

_____

Types of adult illnesses I experienced: _____

_____

Blood Type: _____ Allergies: _____

_____

Weight: _____ Height: _____ Eyeglasses: _____

Surgeries: _____

Age When Died: _____ Date of Death: _____

Cause of Death: _____

_____

Where buried: _____

_____

Children: _____

_____

_____

Full Name: _____

Maiden Name: _____

Date of Birth: _____

Place of Birth: _____

Types of childhood illnesses I experienced: _____
_____

Types of adult illnesses I experienced: _____
_____

Blood Type: _____   Allergies: _____
_____

Weight: _____   Height: _____   Eyeglasses: _____

Surgeries: _____

Age When Died: _____   Date of Death: _____

Cause of Death: _____
_____

Where buried: _____
_____

Children: _____
_____
_____

LINDA CHERYL CONLEY MCCRAY

Full Name: _____

    Maiden Name: _____

Date of Birth: _____

Place of Birth: _____

Types of childhood illnesses I experienced: _____

_____

Types of adult illnesses I experienced: _____

_____

Blood Type: _____ Allergies: _____

_____

Weight: _____ Height: _____ Eyeglasses: _____

Surgeries: _____

Age When Died: _____ Date of Death: _____

Cause of Death: _____

_____

Where buried: _____

_____

Children:_____

_____

_____

Full Name: _____

    Maiden Name: _____

Date of Birth: _____

Place of Birth: _____

Types of childhood illnesses I experienced: _____

_____

Types of adult illnesses I experienced: _____

_____

Blood Type: _____   Allergies: _____

_____

Weight: _____   Height: _____   Eyeglasses: _____

Surgeries: _____

Age When Died: _____   Date of Death: _____

Cause of Death: _____

_____

Where buried: _____

_____

Children: _____

_____

_____

Full Name: _____

    Maiden Name: _____

Date of Birth: _____

Place of Birth: _____

Types of childhood illnesses I experienced: _____

_____

Types of adult illnesses I experienced: _____

_____

Blood Type: _____   Allergies: _____

_____

Weight: _____   Height: _____   Eyeglasses: _____

Surgeries: _____

Age When Died: _____   Date of Death: _____

Cause of Death: _____

_____

Where buried: _____

_____

Children:_____

_____

_____

Full Name: _____

    Maiden Name: _____

Date of Birth: _____

Place of Birth: _____

Types of childhood illnesses I experienced: _____

_____

Types of adult illnesses I experienced: _____

_____

Blood Type: _____   Allergies: _____

_____

Weight: _____   Height: _____   Eyeglasses: _____

Surgeries: _____

Age When Died: _____   Date of Death: _____

Cause of Death: _____

_____

Where buried: _____

_____

Children: _____

_____

_____

Full Name: _____

    Maiden Name: _____

Date of Birth: _____

Place of Birth: _____

Types of childhood illnesses I experienced: _____

_____

Types of adult illnesses I experienced: _____

_____

Blood Type: _____ Allergies: _____

_____

Weight: _____ Height: _____ Eyeglasses: _____

Surgeries: _____

Age When Died: _____ Date of Death: _____

Cause of Death: _____

_____

Where buried: _____

_____

Children: _____

_____

_____

Full Name: _____

    Maiden Name: _____

Date of Birth: _____

Place of Birth: _____

Types of childhood illnesses I experienced: _____

_____

Types of adult illnesses I experienced: _____

_____

Blood Type: _____   Allergies: _____

_____

Weight: _____   Height: _____   Eyeglasses: _____

Surgeries: _____

Age When Died: _____   Date of Death: _____

Cause of Death: _____

_____

Where buried: _____

_____

Children: _____

_____

_____

Full Name: _____

    Maiden Name: _____

Date of Birth: _____

Place of Birth: _____

Types of childhood illnesses I experienced: _____

_____

Types of adult illnesses I experienced: _____

_____

Blood Type: _____   Allergies: _____

_____

Weight: _____   Height: _____   Eyeglasses: _____

Surgeries: _____

Age When Died: _____   Date of Death: _____

Cause of Death: _____

_____

Where buried: _____

_____

Children: _____

_____

_____

Full Name: _____

    Maiden Name: _____

Date of Birth: _____

Place of Birth: _____

Types of childhood illnesses I experienced: _____

_____

Types of adult illnesses I experienced: _____

_____

Blood Type: _____ Allergies: _____

_____

Weight: _____ Height: _____ Eyeglasses: _____

Surgeries: _____

Age When Died: _____ Date of Death: _____

Cause of Death: _____

_____

Where buried: _____

_____

Children: _____

_____

_____

ALL ABOUT MY SPOUSE'S FAMILY

All About My Spouse

Full Name: _____

    Maiden Name: _____

Date of Birth: _____

Place of Birth: _____

Types of childhood illnesses I experienced: _____

_____

Types of adult illnesses I experienced: _____

_____

Blood Type: _____ Allergies: _____

_____

Weight: _____ Height: _____ Eyeglasses: _____

Surgeries: _____

Age When Died: _____ Date of Death: _____

Cause of Death: _____

_____

Where buried: _____

_____

Children: _____

_____

_____

About His/Her Siblings

Full Name: _____

    Maiden Name: _____

Date of Birth: _____

Place of Birth: _____

Types of childhood illnesses I experienced: _____

_____

Types of adult illnesses I experienced: _____

_____

Blood Type: _____ Allergies: _____

_____

Weight: _____ Height: _____ Eyeglasses: _____

Surgeries: _____

Age When Died: _____ Date of Death: _____

Cause of Death: _____

_____

Where buried: _____

_____

Children: _____

_____

_____

Full Name: _____

    Maiden Name: _____

Date of Birth: _____

Place of Birth: _____

Types of childhood illnesses I experienced: _____

_____

Types of adult illnesses I experienced: _____

_____

Blood Type: _____   Allergies: _____

_____

Weight: _____   Height: _____   Eyeglasses: _____

Surgeries: _____

Age When Died: _____   Date of Death: _____

Cause of Death: _____

_____

Where buried: _____

_____

Children: _____

_____

_____

Full Name: _____

   Maiden Name: _____

Date of Birth: _____

Place of Birth: _____

Types of childhood illnesses I experienced: _____

_____

Types of adult illnesses I experienced: _____

_____

Blood Type: _____   Allergies: _____

_____

Weight: _____   Height: _____   Eyeglasses: _____

Surgeries: _____

Age When Died: _____   Date of Death: _____

Cause of Death: _____

_____

Where buried: _____

_____

Children: _____

_____

_____

Full Name: _____

    Maiden Name: _____

Date of Birth: _____

Place of Birth: _____

Types of childhood illnesses I experienced: _____

_____

Types of adult illnesses I experienced: _____

_____

Blood Type: _____ Allergies: _____

_____

Weight: _____ Height: _____ Eyeglasses: _____

Surgeries: _____

Age When Died: _____ Date of Death: _____

Cause of Death: _____

_____

Where buried: _____

_____

Children: _____

_____

_____

Full Name: _____

    Maiden Name: _____

Date of Birth: _____

Place of Birth: _____

Types of childhood illnesses I experienced: _____

_____

Types of adult illnesses I experienced: _____

_____

Blood Type: _____   Allergies: _____

_____

Weight: _____   Height: _____   Eyeglasses: _____

Surgeries: _____

Age When Died: _____   Date of Death: _____

Cause of Death: _____

_____

Where buried: _____

_____

Children: _____

_____

_____

Full Name: _____

    Maiden Name: _____

Date of Birth: _____

Place of Birth: _____

Types of childhood illnesses I experienced: _____

_____

Types of adult illnesses I experienced: _____

_____

Blood Type: _____ Allergies: _____

_____

Weight: _____ Height: _____ Eyeglasses: _____

Surgeries: _____

Age When Died: _____ Date of Death: _____

Cause of Death: _____

_____

Where buried: _____

_____

Children: _____

_____

_____

Full Name: _____

    Maiden Name: _____

Date of Birth: _____

Place of Birth: _____

Types of childhood illnesses I experienced: _____

_____

Types of adult illnesses I experienced: _____

_____

Blood Type: _____ Allergies: _____

_____

Weight: _____ Height: _____ Eyeglasses: _____

Surgeries: _____

Age When Died: _____ Date of Death: _____

Cause of Death: _____

_____

Where buried: _____

_____

Children: _____

_____

_____

LINDA CHERYL CONLEY MCCRAY

Full Name: _____

    Maiden Name: _____

Date of Birth: _____

Place of Birth: _____

Types of childhood illnesses I experienced: _____

_____

Types of adult illnesses I experienced: _____

_____

Blood Type: _____ Allergies: _____

_____

Weight: _____ Height: _____ Eyeglasses: _____

Surgeries: _____

Age When Died: _____ Date of Death: _____

Cause of Death: _____

_____

Where buried: _____

_____

Children: _____

_____

_____

Full Name: _____

    Maiden Name: _____

Date of Birth: _____

Place of Birth: _____

Types of childhood illnesses I experienced: _____

_____

Types of adult illnesses I experienced: _____

_____

Blood Type: _____ Allergies: _____

_____

Weight: _____ Height: _____ Eyeglasses: _____

Surgeries: _____

Age When Died: _____ Date of Death: _____

Cause of Death: _____

_____

Where buried: _____

_____

Children: _____

_____

_____

Full Name: _____

    Maiden Name: _____

Date of Birth: _____

Place of Birth: _____

Types of childhood illnesses I experienced: _____

_____

Types of adult illnesses I experienced: _____

_____

Blood Type: _____ Allergies: _____

_____

Weight: _____ Height: _____ Eyeglasses: _____

Surgeries: _____

Age When Died: _____ Date of Death: _____

Cause of Death: _____

_____

Where buried: _____

_____

Children: _____

_____

_____

ABOUT MY SPOUSE'S MATERNAL FAMILY

About His/Her Mother

Full Name: _____

    Maiden Name: _____

Date of Birth: _____

Place of Birth: _____

Types of childhood illnesses I experienced: _____

_____

Types of adult illnesses I experienced: _____

_____

Blood Type: _____ Allergies: _____

_____

Weight: _____ Height: _____ Eyeglasses: _____

Surgeries: _____

Age When Died: _____ Date of Death: _____

Cause of Death: _____

_____

Where buried: _____

_____

Children: _____

_____

_____

About His/Her Maternal Grandmother

Full Name: _____

    Maiden Name: _____

Date of Birth: _____

Place of Birth: _____

Types of childhood illnesses I experienced: _____

_____

Types of adult illnesses I experienced: _____

_____

Blood Type: _____ Allergies: _____

_____

Weight: _____ Height: _____ Eyeglasses: _____

Surgeries: _____

Age When Died: _____ Date of Death: _____

Cause of Death: _____

_____

Where buried: _____

_____

Children: _____

_____

_____

About His/Her Maternal Grandfather

Full Name: _____

    Maiden Name: _____

Date of Birth: _____

Place of Birth: _____

Types of childhood illnesses I experienced: _____

_____

Types of adult illnesses I experienced: _____

_____

Blood Type: _____ Allergies: _____

_____

Weight: _____ Height: _____ Eyeglasses: _____

Surgeries: _____

Age When Died: _____ Date of Death: _____

Cause of Death: _____

_____

Where buried: _____

_____

Children:_____

_____

_____

About His/Her Mother's Siblings

Full Name: _____

    Maiden Name: _____

Date of Birth: _____

Place of Birth: _____

Types of childhood illnesses I experienced: _____

_____

Types of adult illnesses I experienced: _____

_____

Blood Type: _____   Allergies: _____

_____

Weight: _____   Height: _____   Eyeglasses: _____

Surgeries: _____

Age When Died: _____   Date of Death: _____

Cause of Death: _____

_____

Where buried: _____

_____

Children: _____

_____

_____

Full Name: _____

    Maiden Name: _____

Date of Birth: _____

Place of Birth: _____

Types of childhood illnesses I experienced: _____

_____

Types of adult illnesses I experienced: _____

_____

Blood Type: _____   Allergies: _____

_____

Weight: _____   Height: _____   Eyeglasses: _____

Surgeries: _____

Age When Died: _____   Date of Death: _____

Cause of Death: _____

_____

Where buried: _____

_____

Children:_____

_____

_____

Full Name: _____

    Maiden Name: _____

Date of Birth: _____

Place of Birth: _____

Types of childhood illnesses I experienced: _____

_____

Types of adult illnesses I experienced: _____

_____

Blood Type: _____ Allergies: _____

_____

Weight: _____ Height: _____ Eyeglasses: _____

Surgeries: _____

Age When Died: _____ Date of Death: _____

Cause of Death: _____

_____

Where buried: _____

_____

Children: _____

_____

_____

Full Name: _____

　　　Maiden Name: _____

Date of Birth: _____

Place of Birth: _____

Types of childhood illnesses I experienced: _____

_____

Types of adult illnesses I experienced: _____

_____

Blood Type: _____　　Allergies: _____

_____

Weight: _____　Height: _____　Eyeglasses: _____

Surgeries: _____

Age When Died: _____　　　Date of Death: _____

Cause of Death: _____

_____

Where buried: _____

_____

Children: _____

_____

_____

Full Name: _____

  Maiden Name: _____

Date of Birth: _____

Place of Birth: _____

Types of childhood illnesses I experienced: _____

_____

Types of adult illnesses I experienced: _____

_____

Blood Type: _____   Allergies: _____

_____

Weight: _____   Height: _____   Eyeglasses: _____

Surgeries: _____

Age When Died: _____   Date of Death: _____

Cause of Death: _____

_____

Where buried: _____

_____

Children: _____

_____

_____

Full Name: _____

    Maiden Name: _____

Date of Birth: _____

Place of Birth: _____

Types of childhood illnesses I experienced: _____
_____

Types of adult illnesses I experienced: _____
_____

Blood Type: _____ Allergies: _____
_____

Weight: _____ Height: _____ Eyeglasses: _____

Surgeries: _____

Age When Died: _____ Date of Death: _____

Cause of Death: _____
_____

Where buried: _____
_____

Children: _____
_____
_____

Full Name: _____

    Maiden Name: _____

Date of Birth: _____

Place of Birth: _____

Types of childhood illnesses I experienced: _____
_____

Types of adult illnesses I experienced: _____
_____

Blood Type: _____ Allergies: _____
_____

Weight: _____ Height: _____ Eyeglasses: _____

Surgeries: _____

Age When Died: _____ Date of Death: _____

Cause of Death: _____
_____

Where buried: _____
_____

Children: _____
_____
_____

Full Name: _____

    Maiden Name: _____

Date of Birth: _____

Place of Birth: _____

Types of childhood illnesses I experienced: _____

_____

Types of adult illnesses I experienced: _____

_____

Blood Type: _____ Allergies: _____

_____

Weight: _____ Height: _____ Eyeglasses: _____

Surgeries: _____

Age When Died: _____ Date of Death: _____

Cause of Death: _____

_____

Where buried: _____

_____

Children: _____

_____

_____

Full Name: _____

    Maiden Name: _____

Date of Birth: _____

Place of Birth: _____

Types of childhood illnesses I experienced: _____

_____

Types of adult illnesses I experienced: _____

_____

Blood Type: _____ Allergies: _____

_____

Weight: _____ Height: _____ Eyeglasses: _____

Surgeries: _____

Age When Died: _____ Date of Death: _____

Cause of Death: _____

_____

Where buried: _____

_____

Children: _____

_____

_____

Full Name: _____

    Maiden Name: _____

Date of Birth: _____

Place of Birth: _____

Types of childhood illnesses I experienced: _____

_____

Types of adult illnesses I experienced: _____

_____

Blood Type: _____ Allergies: _____

_____

Weight: _____ Height: _____ Eyeglasses: _____

Surgeries: _____

Age When Died: _____ Date of Death: _____

Cause of Death: _____

_____

Where buried: _____

_____

Children: _____

_____

_____

Full Name: _____

    Maiden Name: _____

Date of Birth: _____

Place of Birth: _____

Types of childhood illnesses I experienced: _____

_____

Types of adult illnesses I experienced: _____

_____

Blood Type: _____ Allergies: _____

_____

Weight: _____ Height: _____ Eyeglasses: _____

Surgeries: _____

Age When Died: _____ Date of Death: _____

Cause of Death: _____

_____

Where buried: _____

_____

Children: _____

_____

_____

LINDA CHERYL CONLEY MCCRAY

ABOUT MY SPOUSE'S PATERNAL FAMILY

About His/Her Father

Full Name: _____

Maiden Name: _____

Date of Birth: _____

Place of Birth: _____

Types of childhood illnesses I experienced: _____
_____

Types of adult illnesses I experienced: _____
_____

Blood Type: _____ Allergies: _____
_____

Weight: _____ Height: _____ Eyeglasses: _____

Surgeries: _____

Age When Died: _____ Date of Death: _____

Cause of Death: _____
_____

Where buried: _____
_____

Children: _____
_____
_____

About His/Her Paternal Grandmother

Full Name: _____

    Maiden Name: _____

Date of Birth: _____

Place of Birth: _____

Types of childhood illnesses I experienced: _____

_____

Types of adult illnesses I experienced: _____

_____

Blood Type: _____ Allergies: _____

_____

Weight: _____ Height: _____ Eyeglasses: _____

Surgeries: _____

Age When Died: _____ Date of Death: _____

Cause of Death: _____

_____

Where buried: _____

_____

Children: _____

_____

_____

About His/Her Paternal Grandfather

Full Name: _____

    Maiden Name: _____

Date of Birth: _____

Place of Birth: _____

Types of childhood illnesses I experienced: _____

_____

Types of adult illnesses I experienced: _____

_____

Blood Type: _____ Allergies: _____

_____

Weight: _____ Height: _____ Eyeglasses: _____

Surgeries: _____

Age When Died: _____ Date of Death: _____

Cause of Death: _____

_____

Where buried: _____

_____

Children: _____

_____

_____

About His/Her Father's Siblings

Full Name: _____

    Maiden Name: _____

Date of Birth: _____

Place of Birth: _____

Types of childhood illnesses I experienced: _____
_____

Types of adult illnesses I experienced: _____
_____

Blood Type: _____ Allergies: _____
_____

Weight: _____ Height: _____ Eyeglasses: _____

Surgeries: _____

Age When Died: _____ Date of Death: _____

Cause of Death: _____
_____

Where buried: _____
_____

Children: _____
_____
_____

Full Name: _____

    Maiden Name: _____

Date of Birth: _____

Place of Birth: _____

Types of childhood illnesses I experienced: _____

_____

Types of adult illnesses I experienced: _____

_____

Blood Type: _____ Allergies: _____

_____

Weight: _____ Height: _____ Eyeglasses: _____

Surgeries: _____

Age When Died: _____ Date of Death: _____

Cause of Death: _____

_____

Where buried: _____

_____

Children:_____

_____

_____

Full Name: _____

    Maiden Name: _____

Date of Birth: _____

Place of Birth: _____

Types of childhood illnesses I experienced: _____

_____

Types of adult illnesses I experienced: _____

_____

Blood Type: _____ Allergies: _____

_____

Weight: _____ Height: _____ Eyeglasses: _____

Surgeries: _____

Age When Died: _____ Date of Death: _____

Cause of Death: _____

_____

Where buried: _____

_____

Children: _____

_____

_____

Full Name: _____

    Maiden Name: _____

Date of Birth: _____

Place of Birth: _____

Types of childhood illnesses I experienced: _____

_____

Types of adult illnesses I experienced: _____

_____

Blood Type: _____ Allergies: _____

_____

Weight: _____ Height: _____ Eyeglasses: _____

Surgeries: _____

Age When Died: _____ Date of Death: _____

Cause of Death: _____

_____

Where buried: _____

_____

Children: _____

_____

_____

Full Name: _____

    Maiden Name: _____

Date of Birth: _____

Place of Birth: _____

Types of childhood illnesses I experienced: _____

_____

Types of adult illnesses I experienced: _____

_____

Blood Type: _____   Allergies: _____

_____

Weight: _____   Height: _____   Eyeglasses: _____

Surgeries: _____

Age When Died: _____   Date of Death: _____

Cause of Death: _____

_____

Where buried: _____

_____

Children: _____

_____

_____

Full Name: _____

   Maiden Name: _____

Date of Birth: _____

Place of Birth: _____

Types of childhood illnesses I experienced: _____
_____

Types of adult illnesses I experienced: _____
_____

Blood Type: _____   Allergies: _____
_____

Weight: _____   Height: _____   Eyeglasses: _____

Surgeries: _____

Age When Died: _____   Date of Death: _____

Cause of Death: _____
_____

Where buried: _____
_____

Children:_____
_____
_____

Full Name: _____

   Maiden Name: _____

Date of Birth: _____

Place of Birth: _____

Types of childhood illnesses I experienced: _____

_____

Types of adult illnesses I experienced: _____

_____

Blood Type: _____ Allergies: _____

_____

Weight: _____ Height: _____ Eyeglasses: _____

Surgeries: _____

Age When Died: _____ Date of Death: _____

Cause of Death: _____

_____

Where buried: _____

_____

Children: _____

_____

_____

Full Name: _____

    Maiden Name: _____

Date of Birth: _____

Place of Birth: _____

Types of childhood illnesses I experienced: _____

_____

Types of adult illnesses I experienced: _____

_____

Blood Type: _____ Allergies: _____

_____

Weight: _____ Height: _____ Eyeglasses: _____

Surgeries: _____

Age When Died: _____ Date of Death: _____

Cause of Death: _____

_____

Where buried: _____

_____

Children: _____

_____

_____

Full Name: _____

    Maiden Name: _____

Date of Birth: _____

Place of Birth: _____

Types of childhood illnesses I experienced: _____

_____

Types of adult illnesses I experienced: _____

_____

Blood Type: _____ Allergies: _____

_____

Weight: _____ Height: _____ Eyeglasses: _____

Surgeries: _____

Age When Died: _____ Date of Death: _____

Cause of Death: _____

_____

Where buried: _____

_____

Children:_____

_____

_____

Full Name: _____

    Maiden Name: _____

Date of Birth: _____

Place of Birth: _____

Types of childhood illnesses I experienced: _____

_____

Types of adult illnesses I experienced: _____

_____

Blood Type: _____ Allergies: _____

_____

Weight: _____ Height: _____ Eyeglasses: _____

Surgeries: _____

Age When Died: _____ Date of Death: _____

Cause of Death: _____

_____

Where buried: _____

_____

Children: _____

_____

_____

STORIES THAT TOUCHED MY LIFE

Expressing Myself!!

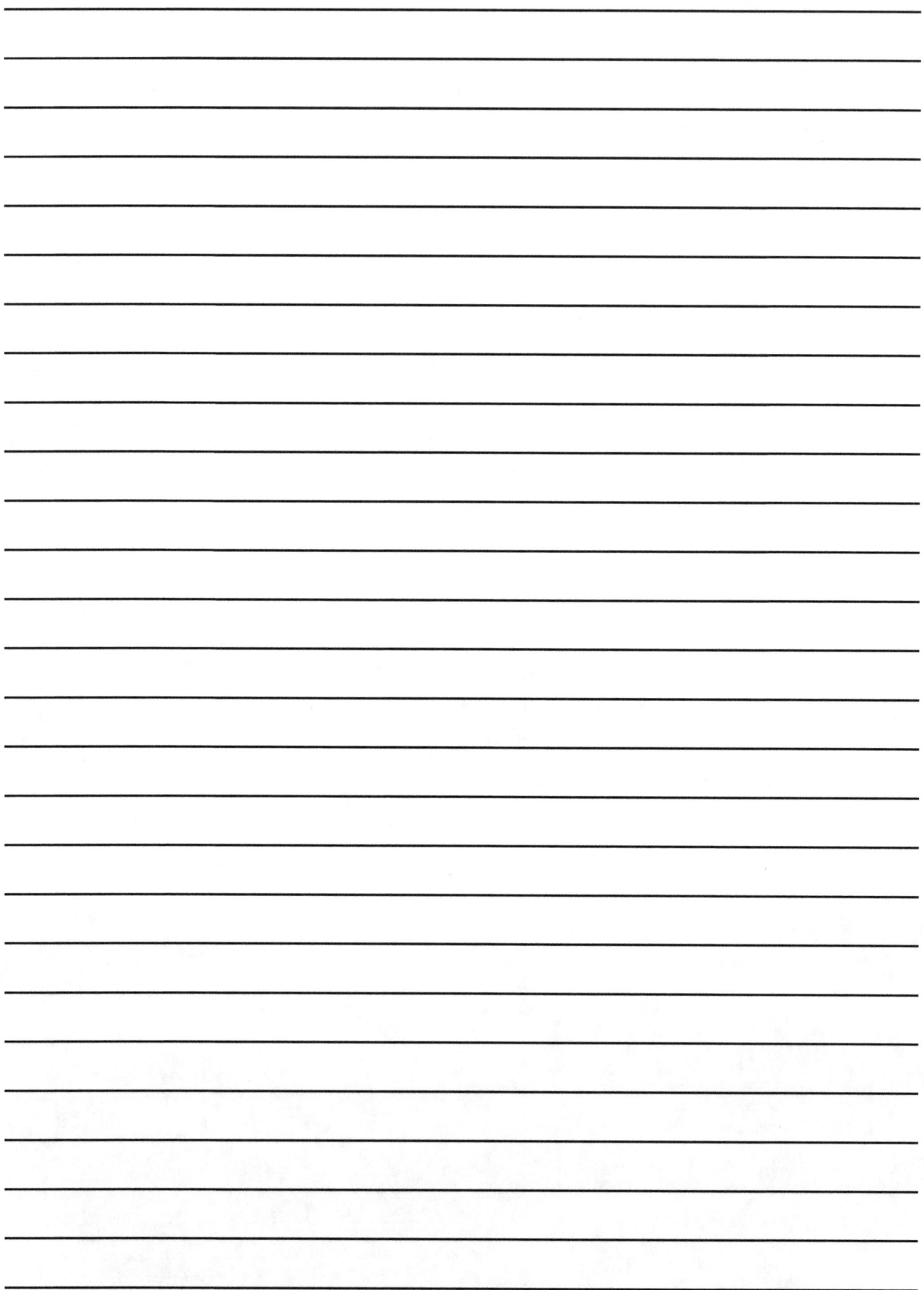

www.ingramcontent.com/pod-product-compliance
Lightning Source LLC
Chambersburg PA
CBHW080420030426
42335CB00020B/2519

* 9 7 8 1 9 5 5 9 4 4 6 0 1 *